FPL

Functional Personal Lifestyle

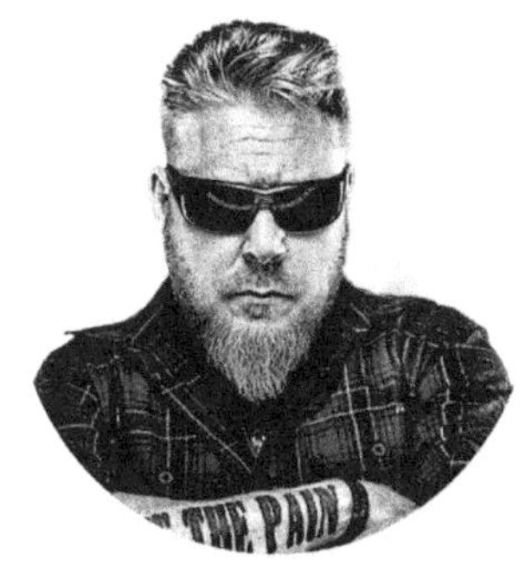

BOONE CUTLER PROTOCOLS

BOONE CUTLER
with GEOFF DARDIA

ATTRIBUTIONS

Editor: Boone Cutler
Cover Design & Typesetting: Robbie Grayson III
Interior Text: EB Garamond

BOOK PUBLISHING INFORMATION

Traitmarker Books
www.traitmarkerbooks.com

traitmarker@gmail.com

NOTE

TO THE BAD MOTHERFUCKER READING THIS

Get a pen and circle the phrase "It still works" every time you see it. You'll see why later. This volume exposes the reader to numerous Warfighter health issues. Not every reader has the same issues, so examine the principles that work for your personal situation. Write in the book. It works. *It still works.*

BOONE CUTLER | July 2020

NATIONAL SUICIDE PREVENTION HOTLINE

1-800-273-8255

FPL

Functional Personal Lifestyle
by BOONE CUTLER

1

I'm not a doctor. I'm a Warfighter that has died and then lived. I spent two years in the hospital after my time in war, and since then I've learned a lot. This is my journey... so far.

2

In 2006, Walter Reed was a chemical prison to me. I was on every drug that killed model Anna Nicole Smith, I was on every drug that killed actor Heath Ledger, and I was on every drug that was slowly killing me. I overdosed dozens of times, and at night I'd commonly awaken puking what looked like coffee grounds. Too many drugs to manage with TBI. It didn't work. It was a bad idea.

3

Chloral-hydrate, promethazine, zolpidem, nortriptyline, morphine, divalproex, hydrocodone, metoprolol, prazosin, ibuprofen, diazepam, lorazepam, topamax, quetiapine, meperidine, trazodone, mirtazapine, hydromorphone, and more were mostly being foolishly self-administered while I was having serious cognitive and memory deficits caused from a blast injury that left me with moderate traumatic brain injury.

4

Two years of drugs (Combat-cocktail with Zombie Dope) from Walter Reed followed me to the Veterans Administration hospital after I was discharged. I wasn't better… I was worse but I complained less about my problems like a good zombie should. Not much worked.

5

I stayed suicidal and the anger grew as the slut captivated me. Confusion and sadness were a reprieve. "War porn" on YouTube was my favorite pastime because I just wanted to go back to war. I obsessed over videos from war. I was homesick for war. It was a deep longing for the life I missed. War. It was the last place I felt comfortable. War. *War.* War. My addictions to the meds grew worse as they became less effective. Less zombie and more Hulk happened. NyQuil™ and a good amount of Scotch were how I dealt with it... on top of taking the meds. It didn't work.

6

My mistress was in control of me. All the drug addictions made suicide my ultimate fantasy as she whispered, *The world will be better without you... People don't care... Only the children are innocent, everything else deserves to be killed - one way or another... After the first one, the rest are just numbers... Killing yourself is the one death you'll never have to mourn... Fuck it, turn in to the pylon... Eat all the meds, have a few drinks, and go to sleep.* My mind was an instrument for her to play, and the drugs created histrionic delusions that she used to entice me to kill myself.

7

Lockdown. I ended up locked-down.

8

Hourly bed checks and more drugs. Inpatient. Psych ward 101 and lots of accusations from the staff that I couldn't remember, all because of Zombie dope. I was totally defenseless, and that changed things. Reality woke me from a long stupor.

9

Being defenseless was my worst nightmare, and I wanted personal control back no matter what the cost. The drugs had to stop.

10

They tried to medicate me more and I refused. They threatened me... I still refused. I went AMA (Against Medical Advice) and refused the Zombie Dope. Seventeen days later, I was released and I was 70% clean. They also determined that my hormone levels were very low. I started hormone replacement. It worked. It still works.

11

I dropped the Zombie dope but not the opiates. Better, yes- but far from good. I was eating 30 mg of Morphine with 70 mg of Oxycontin daily when I eventually stopped... but "eventually" was still years away. No lie... pain hurts and chronic pain was an issue I couldn't kick. I still can't... but I've learned a few things that work.

12

Nightly marijuana use replaced all the Zombie Dope. I learned that if I could get good sleep, I could cope. Marijuana was a blessing. Sure, I broke the law. Fuck 'em. I was alive. Nightmares and regrets became manageable. The guilt monster got a leash that I controlled, and the slut learned to shut her mouth. It turned out that a lot of my psych issues were insomnia and hormone-related. Many Warfighters have the same issues. Hormones and weed was a better option over psych meds. It worked. It still works.

13

My injury list from my Paratrooper lifestyle is long: 7 knee surgeries, 6 shoulder surgeries, back surgery, traction from a C1/C2 subluxation, heavy metal toxicity, brain damage from numerous concussions and high order explosives... the list goes on. This is common in my community. Our medical records are volumes long.

14

Our pain is the residue of our service.

15

Being willing to die is literally in the Warfighter job description, and we are willing to die so we can kill for the benefit of others.

16

Best damn job I ever had.

17

Getting off the opiates was the next mission... easier said than done. I wasn't sure when or if it would happen: chronic pain... the mean bitch that is always waiting to remind you of a bad situation.

18

Here's the trick though... managing the chemical dependency. I had to detox a few times a year just so I could start back at a lower dose to keep pain meds working. Detoxing really pissed off the mean bitch of chronic pain.

19

OPIOID DETOX. Shakes, unremitting migraines, puking, endless dry heaves, hot-cold-hot-cold flashes, depression, and sadness. That's what I had to do a few times a year to keep that mean bitch off my back. Words can't explain what it's really like. Opiates always become a torturous tether to insanity.

20

Once the detox was over, I stayed off opiates for as long as I could until I couldn't. The mean bitch never stops and chronic pain is a mean bitch.

21

Opiates continued. And so did the addiction cycle.

22

My brother, Nacho, called. We both knew the same slut. Suicide affected us both, but neither of us knew it about each other. Same with my other brother, Hickey. The slut was sneaky, and she was fucking everyone I knew. We had all flirted with Suicide and never told each other.

23

The Spartan Pledge began immediately, and it gave us all a new platform for understanding, brotherhood, and it gave us a plan. It was the battle drill for what to do when we didn't know what to do. It worked. It still works.

24

THE SPARTAN PLEDGE

I will not take my own life by my own hand until I talk to my battle buddy first. My mission is to find a mission to help my Warfighter Family. This is how the histrionic delusions lose their power.

25

The three things a leader must provide are purpose, direction, and motivation. *The Spartan Pledge* gave us those three things, and that's how we found our common ethos again. The common ethos is the thing that makes us all "want to go back to war." It worked. It still works.

26

Opiates continued and kidney disease started. Blood pressure got worse and harder to control. Migraines were even more frequent. I'd vomit daily, and the Tijuana trots were more like the Kentucky Derby for years and years. Gut issues are no joke.

27

Degenerative brain disease from TBI. I was diagnosed Parkinson's or Parkinsonism in 2014. It was rough. Dystonia was my "Warfighter Smile" but marijuana helped and the doc was awesomely supportive of cannabinoid-therapy rather than fearful. I'd had undiagnosed Parkinson's since the war. It was missed. I began using marijuana for Parkinsonism flare-ups ... it worked. It still works.

28

Opiates continued. Switching between opiates and changing combinations of opiates used together became a thing. Bottles as big as footballs.

29

Cannabidiol (CBD) came on the scene and I walked off the opiates after, dare I say, a decade-ish long battle. CBD was also great for social anxiety that was most definitely a problem. I never liked being in public high so I didn't do it but CBD was all the help I needed without the high. The mean bitch of chronic pain took a chill-pill. It works. It still works.

30

Finally, I was no longer addicted to anything and immediately my mistress slut of suicide was no longer my daily visitor. She still lived around the corner, but the frequent booty-calls we're finally over.

31

Chronic pain, suicidal ideation, insomnia, and Parkinson's were all being mitigated by some form of cannabinoid therapy. It worked. It still works.

32

I learned that stress is accumulative. The more you have, the less you can take. If your bench press max is 185 pounds, that's it. Stress is the same. Once you are maxed, that's it. Only time and training can increase your max. And it has to be balanced.

33

Ever seen someone bench 185 pounds with 135 pounds on one side and 50 on the other? Sounds ridiculous, but that's what it's like trying to balance

TBI and PTSD with life while on all the drugs and dealing with addiction.

34

I was able to start finding balance: first with *The Spartan Pledge* and then with the help of cannabinoids. And none of it would have been possible without a caregiver.

35

If you have TBI with cognitive disorder and memory impairment… you need a caregiver on some level to make sure you don't burn down the house from leaving the stove on, and at least so that someone with a memory can relay accurate info to and from the doctor so you don't fuck yourself more. This is what works. Work as a team. It still works.

36

My wife is amazing. Having someone that can remember the path to progress and avoid repeating past mistakes is invaluable. This is an imperative. It still works.

37

I thought I'd try light exercise and a better diet to make myself better. A daily workout routine got easier over time, and it helped with pain control. A low sugar, organic, high protein diet made me feel better. It worked. It still works.

38

My first cardiac incident happened. Damn. Those years on drugs hurt my kidneys badly. The decade of diarrhea didn't help, and a Prednisone shot from a procedure left me with critically low potassium that was near-fatal.

39

We adjusted and drove on. My blood pressure got even worse over time. We tried everything to no avail.

40

Living the ethos inspired by *The Spartan Pledge,* cannabinoids, daily exercise, and a healthful diet worked. It still works.

41

The Shoulder Debacle of 2017. They were pumping very strong antibiotics directly into my heart to save my life because of an infection from a service-connected shoulder surgery. It took a lot to repair my shoulder, and it all had to be undone. They pulled out all the screws and cut off the dead flesh. Four surgeries later, it was worse than when they started.

42

Over nearly a year, we adjusted and drove on, minus a chunk of rabid meat they cut out of my arm. Exercise got harder, but I'm creative. Fuck it: I wasn't planning on winning Mr. Universe anyway. Again, cannabinoids get a solid high five. I never craved opiates for pain control through it all. It worked. It still works.

43

Maintaining the things that worked got me better faster and kept my spirits up. I didn't have a pity-party over it, I was happy that they saved my arm and I didn't die. It took all of 2018 to recover. Keep what works and keep doing that. It still works.

44

September 2018. I was at death's door again, and this time I brought a breach kit. The years of uncontrollable blood pressure and the strong antibiotics they pumped into my heart the year before after the shoulder infection were no joke. My heart gave out. We missed something, and I was on a ride down the death spiral. Cardiomyopathy, heart failure, and polycythemia all at the same time and the bad kidneys didn't help. Down... down... down. I was no-shit dying. What did we miss?

45

My heart was enlarged and no longer wanted to beat. My injection fraction was 30% and my organs were struggling. Within six months, I'd be taking a dirt nap and there was no way around it.

46

Just about the time I figured out how not to want to

die everyday, I was dying. Go figure. Call Alanis Morissette because that was fucking ironic.

47

The deathbed is filled with reflection in the midst of anger and denial. I've nearly-died a lot in my life, but it was more like realizing what happened after it was over. When you have experienced war, you have experienced somebody who is shooting at you and who missed you but you didn't miss them... then the threat is over. Good marksmanship and a 5.56mm projectile traveling 2970 feet per second solve the problem. But dying from a heart condition... that's a whole different kind of dying. It makes you wait and feel life slip as you slowly and simply "go dim." Not easy.

48

After all my wife had been through to get me well, one issue at a time had led to this. I'd catch her crying. She tried to be brave for me and hide it but I knew. We told the kids the truth. It's better that way. It was not easy. What did we miss that got me here?

49

From my deathbed, I learned what was important about life, and I saw my family pull together as a team to cover down on what needed to be done without me. I've never been prouder than I was when I saw their character and training come together for a common cause without my leading them. I don't think anything could make a man prouder than that. This is the biggest blessing of my life.

50

But what caused it all? What did we miss? Well, remember the brain damage? Here's how brain damage becomes a heart problem: I had undiagnosed Central Sleep Apnea which is secondary to brain damage. Everyone with brain damage most likely has some level of Central Sleep Apnea. Not Obstructive Sleep Apnea but CENTRAL SLEEP APNEA. Unfortunately, I learned that too late. We missed it.

51

Central Sleep Apnea is when the brain isn't telling the body to breathe adequately during sleep. A person with Central Sleep Apnea must have a machine to regulate breathing at night, and there's zero way around it. OBSTRUCTIVE Sleep Apnea can be corrected but CENTRAL Sleep Apnea can not, so long as the person has brain damage. I had probably needed a machine to help me breathe when I slept since the time I was injured in Iraq from a mortar explosion and I never knew it.

52

My uncontrollable blood pressure was a sign that my heart and brain were starving for oxygen while I was sleeping. Always being tired was a sign, too. And had I gotten a sleep study, it would have been diagnosed.

53

Hypoxia kills. If you have TBI, get a sleep study or you will die a shitty death and you'll have to helplessly watch your family suffer watching you slowly die in front of them.

54

My wife and kids never lost their bearing or composure in my presence. They were trained to be this way. We handle the mission first and cry later if we need to. The Great Santini couldn't be prouder. And I cried alone, too, so I wouldn't upset them.

55

I didn't cry for me, but I cried for their controlled anguish and for the times I knew I wouldn't be around for. Soon, I would never again make love to my wife or enjoy Sunday family dinner, and never would I walk my girls down the aisle or mentor my sons through fatherhood. And I was seemingly destined to be a myth to my future grandkids. Like Bruce Lee but with sunglasses and a cool beard.

56

Life is a game within a game of games. We wear masks and we remove them. Nobody picks our masks for us. The time for joy is in-the-moment. Joy can't be banked for later, it's a NOW thing. Enjoy the games, every chance you get while you can still play and make

sure you have a happy-mask somewhere in your
kitbag.

57

Enjoy joy, now, or you never will. Don't die joyless.

58

And then angels appeared. An amazing woman
reached out to me that had lost her oldest son, a
veteran, to pharmacologically induced suicide and
then her other son took his own life because he was so
lost and heartbroken over his brother. She told me
about how she couldn't save her sons but she was
going to save me. Her name is Mama Lutz.

59

A friend at *Warfighter Hemp* also reached out and
contributed. His name is Steven "Luker" Danyluk.

60

Between these two titans in the Warfighter
Community, they paid a lot of money for me to stay

alive with Hyperbaric Oxygen Therapy until I could get to Panama for Stem Cell therapy. They paid for all of it. Nearly $50K. None of this is covered by insurance, and we weren't 100% sure it would even help. We also didn't know if I'd survive waiting for the appointment.

61

We waited from October to January, and in the meantime my wife carted me to HyperBaric Oxygen Therapy (HBOT) everyday so we could try to get pressurized oxygen into my brain and organs and help me breathe. My breathing was so labored that I couldn't stand and brush my teeth without becoming breathless and by this time I couldn't drive anymore.

62

We got the sleep study and a machine to help me breathe while I slept. My Central Sleep Apnea was severe. My breathing stopping on an average of 70 times per hour for more than 10 seconds at a time was a nightly event before the machine. People who bitch about getting a sleep study or say they can't stand the machine at night must have had easy lives because it's totally doable. The new technology is a quiet machine and a ton of different masks to choose from. Stop being a bitch if you are putting it off. Think of it as a supercharger for a sex machine.

63

Let all the air out of your lungs and count to 15: see how you feel. Try it 70 times in an hour... hour after hour. Hypoxia kills.

64

Once a Warfighter gets past the insomnia, night sweats and nightmares... they might think they are sleeping but they might not be because if they have TBI, they are suffocating. All. Night. Long. Year after year.

65

My wife and I flew all the way to Panama City, Panama and by that time I was so weak that my wife pushed me in a wheelchair. Humbling as fuck for a guy that once ran two miles in under eleven minutes. Mortality sucks when you feel it.

66

It is a life changing experience, being forced into a wheelchair. If I ever see someone treating a person in a wheelchair like they are "in the way" - I'll beat their ass. Just trying to order food in an airport when people were in a hurry around me has shown me just how shitty people can be. None of them would have pulled that shit with me standing but seated, sick, in a wheelchair they felt justified to treat me like I was furniture that was in the wrong place. Completely dismissive of simple respect.

67

The Stem Cell Institute in Panama saved my life. The night following the first day of therapy was like some transformative Wolverine shit on a molecular level. I could feel my body's systems re-booting and it hurt in unusual ways but it only got better and better. It worked. It still works.

68

Months passed. My heart recovered. I recovered. It worked. It still works.

69

From the stem cells my brain damage somewhat improved. Cognitively anyhow. And though my memory didn't improve, my ability to understand how bad my memory is has improved, that was a shock and a plus. Cognitive impairment impairs a person's ability to assess the severity of their own health. Wow. Helluva realization, but it's true. If you have cognitive disorder - you truly NEED a caregiver. It works. It still works.

70

Let's Review. Living the ethos of the Spartan Pledge (where's your battle buddy and what is your mission) Cannabinoids (not just THC, but the other cannabinoids too), Hormone replacement, Hyperbaric Oxygen Therapy, CPAP Machine to breathe during sleep, sensible exercise, a balanced low sugar / high protein / organic diet, stem cell therapy and now Human Growth Hormone. This is a mixed bag that combines with my FPL... Functional Personalized Lifestyle. You need to establish your FPL. It works. It still works.

71

THE FPL... Functional Personalized Lifestyle is healthy medicine and it's your FINAL PROTECTIVE LINE against dysfunctional lifestyles and bad medicine. Geoff Dardia, the founder of SOF (Special Operations Forces) Health Initiatives, is the guru of all things functional-medicine in the Warfighter Community. We've been buddied-up for nearly a decade and knowledge from our journeys and mutual learning have been spread far and wide. He's a genius. It worked. It still works.

72

My journey is not unique, but my outcome is. Too many of us have "mysteriously" died in our sleep at a young age, taken our own lives, died from service-connected cancer, angrily plowed vehicles into trees and pylons, hoping to be done with it all.

73

Brain injuries have been mistreated as if they were psych issues. We can't talk our way out of brain damage with a psychologist, and psych meds are a foolish remedy for TBI. We've been denied the medicine and modalities that work. We've also been personally irresponsible with our lack of discipline to take care of personal health.

74

Heavy metal toxicity, mefloquine toxicity, poisoning from burn pits, and living in areas of the world that are simply contaminated from decades of war and uranium exposure are real issues, and they are the issues that need more attention.

75

We overcome what we overcome when we coalesce as a group, motivate each other with accountability and share the information about what works. It works. It still works.

76

Design your own FPL... smartly. It works. Keep it updated and you'll be able to say... it still works.

NATIONAL SUICIDE PREVENTION HOTLINE

1-800-273-8255

WHAT IS YOUR FUNCTIONAL PERSONALIZED LIFESTYLE?

*A Brief Overview of Protocols
That Might Work for You*

(Research, add, delete, and personalize)

CANNABINOIDS

Indica strains of Marijuana with THC are good for insomnia when CBD isn't strong enough. THC is great for insomnia and some chronic pain. CBD helps with inflammation, and pain comes from inflammation. CBD also helps with insomnia for many people, and it's known to lower blood pressure, treat anxiety, and help with brain disease. Edibles and flower are the safest forms. Water pipes work well. A couple rounds for three to six weeks of RSO (Rick Simpson Oil) per year are great for wellness.

HBOT (Hyperbaric Oxygen Therapy):

Great for brain injuries and wound healing. If you have TBI, HBOT is helpful to a lot of people.

HORMONE REPLACEMENT

If your hormones aren't right; you aren't right. Get your hormones checked and see if you need supplementation. Even Human Growth Hormone (Norditropin) is now covered by TRICARE for Warfighters with TBI.

SLEEP STUDY

If you snore or if you've had a brain injury, get a sleep study. It's 1000x easier than you think it is. Don't avoid it.

SENSIBLE EXERCISE

If you aren't on active duty, learn to do PT like a civilian. Long term sustainability and health is the new mission. Yoga is probably better for you than running and will burn the calories you need burned. Go rock climbing with a Warfighter group like GallantFew.org who have groups and trips year-round. Mountain biking, weightlifting, cycling, swimming, diving, hiking, and maybe some group sponsored occasional road marches are options to explore. Team RWB has a great reputation for exercise activities. Find the sustainable activities for your current lifestyle.

STEM CELLS

All stem cell therapy works. Efficacy depends on getting the correct number of healthy cells that you need. Make sure you select a reputable doctor, and remember that some therapies aren't done in the United States. Most of the best therapy is only offered abroad.

ALTERNATIVE DRUG THERAPY

The truth is that DMT, LSD, MDMA, and psilocybin are either already FDA-approved or will soon be approved. It's not your grandpa's hippy trip either. Ketamine is also becoming popular with many. What guys tell me is that it's like a reset button for the brain. I've never done any of these therapies, but the people I know that have swear by it.

NUTRITION

Make your weight normal, avoid sugar, and find the nutrition plan that works best for your goals. Intermediate fasting is becoming very popular and worth researching.

TAKE *THE SPARTAN PLEDGE*

Live by an ethos again. *A Warfighter with a mission is a deadly Warfighter but a Warfighter without a mission is a dead Warfighter.* Find your mission or die... without one.

LIFESTYLE

Avoid prolonged self-isolation, and make sure you help others. Warfighters need an element of selfless service in their lives, and that's how we help ourselves. I recommend finding a local Buddy-Up meeting sponsored by the *LCpl Janos V. Lutz Foundation.* Warrior Pointe also has meetings and is a good place to hang out. Irreverent Warriors is a good group to be a part of. Bottom line is, *Find a Warfighter group to coalesce with.*

ADDICTIONS

Deal with them NOW. Contact American Addiction Centers. It's either low or no cost for Warfighters, and my buddy Dan Cerrillo is a head honcho there so I know it's good.

COUNSELING

It works for a lot of people. If you need to remain anonymous, contact giveanhour.org for free and anonymous counseling. Otherwise, the VetCenter is in every major city for Warfighters that served in combat and counseling is also available for their family members at no cost.

CAREGIVER

If you have TBI, you probably need a Caregiver at least to help keep the meds straight and to recall information from and to your medical provider. Having a Caregiver that you choose is part of the medical plan. Look into the V.A. Comprehensive Caregiver Program.

NEUROMUSCULAR CALIBRATION

Calibration is the ultimate reset for the body and brain to recover from Trauma(s). Precise movements called "Calibrations" are performed during a series of sessions to cause the brain to go into a light trance - the optimum state for the nervous system to restore its original setting(s) or to be optimized. The result is a sustained, calm, mental and physical functioning and optimum breathing. This leads to better sleep, clearer thinking, more confidence, stabilized emotions, substantially reduced body pain, and overall better health.

FINAL THOUGHT

The terms "Shell Shock" and "Soldier's Heart" were accurate terms even before both could be proven with adequate medical explanation. Then the medical establishment used the wrong term, and ... ugh.

The brain damage from explosions affects the body and BRAIN function. First it affects behavior, and then the brain damage (AKA TBI) causes Central Sleep Apnea and (maybe) Parkinsonism and other conditions caused by degenerative brain disease from TBI.

Few of us were ever told what our TBIs might result in. Some result in poor health and cardiomyopathy from the lack of oxygen during sleep from Central Sleep Apnea. The heart rapidly dies under these conditions, and the brain remains oxygen-starved. And that's what a "Soldier's Heart" is.

Medical science did not help us when they lumped everything under the psychiatric diagnosis of Post Traumatic Stress Disorder (PTSD).

Warfighters need neurological advances and treatment rather than more shrinks and psych meds.

Stop treating TBI as a psychiatric disorder. And if you have TBI, get a sleep study.

#StemCells4ShellShock

HOW FUNCTIONAL MEDICINE CAME TO THE MILITARY

by COURTNEY HELGOE |
January-February2020

Master Sergeant Geoff Dardia has a no-legs plan.

He's served as a U.S. Army Green Beret since 2004. If he loses his legs to an explosion or gunfire, he's prepared to build his own "robot legs" so he can stay on active duty. This is something he learned from his Special Operations colleague Chuck, who served for 10 years on a leg he designed himself. Because of the deep trust Dardia shares with his fellow soldiers, he says he sleeps better on deployment — even when that means lying under a truck, in the field, protected only by his mates — than he does back home.

The no-legs strategy isn't his only contingency plan. After a set of mysterious symptoms nearly forced his retirement in 2012, Dardia began to arm himself with a wealth of health knowledge that has allowed him to keep serving. Today, he and a growing number of forward-thinking military healthcare providers are working to expand access to unconventional, person-centered healthcare in the military. If they're successful, they may help prove that a whole-person approach to health is the best tool for treating those who serve — and for the rest of us, too.

FORCE MULTIPLIER

Dardia was first deployed to Afghanistan in 2005. After three successful tours, he was selected to work stateside as an instructor in a specialized advanced-urban-combat school. The job involved spending several hours each day and night in indoor shoot houses or outdoor ranges, breathing in a toxic mix of heavy metals from munitions and explosives.

By 2011 he began experiencing a mysterious set of symptoms: fatigue, migraines, short-term memory loss, vision problems, brain fog, weight gain, no libido. Itchy rashes appeared on his legs. And though he was just 31, his hair was graying and falling out. His exercise and eating habits hadn't changed, but everything else had. "I'm dragging a dead body here," he told his doctor.

His symptoms confounded his healthcare providers. Aside from fatigue, they couldn't offer a firm diagnosis, much less a solution. He was repeatedly told that his condition was all in his head. Some suggested PTSD, others depression. That didn't feel right;

Dardia loves his job. "The only thing I'm depressed about is not being able to do what I used to do," he told them.

In the absence of a diagnosis, Dardia began approaching his condition as he'd been trained: He studied his environment. "What I do as a Special Forces operator is look at the threats in the environment and how they impact my operation. It's not just me. You know, How do I interact with my environment?"

He began reading medical journals. "I got obsessed with what was killing me," he says. He learned that his symptoms matched those of neurotoxicity and discovered what types of diagnostic testing he needed. Everything pointed to heavy-metal poisoning, as well as traumatic brain injury (TBI) and an adverse reaction to antimalarial medications.

In 2012 Dardia was finally referred for a comprehensive TBI evaluation at a high-level military hospital. His providers determined that in addition to brain injury, he had severe binocular-vision disorder (a condition in which the eyes stop working as a team), hormone dysfunction and fertility issues, leaky gut, a lesion on his pituitary gland, and white-matter lesions on his brain.

These issues were not just bad luck. Dardia had been

exposed to millions of rounds of ammunition, countless explosions, and thousands of explosive charges during his military training and career.

In 2013 he and another soldier with similar symptoms met with Kevin Dorrance, chief of internal medicine at Walter Reed National Military Medical Center. Dorrance suspected lead poisoning in both men and administered bone-lead x-rays. The scans showed the two soldiers were "packed" with the toxic mineral.

One might assume that combat represents the greatest existential threat to military personnel, but most face a range of health hazards that are far less visible.

By then Dardia had begun volunteering for the Task Force Dagger Foundation (TFD), a Dallas-based nonprofit that offers support to injured Special Operations members. He knew that plenty of his fellow service members faced complex symptoms like his, so he created a program for TFD to offer "next-generation health solutions" to other Special Operations Forces (SOF) and their families.

After returning from another tour in Afghanistan in 2015, Dardia, with the help of TFD, went to Cleveland Clinic's Center for Functional Medicine to seek treatment.

"One of the major blind spots of conventional medicine is heavy-metal toxicity," says Mark Hyman, MD, who treated Dardia at the Cleveland Clinic. "Heavy metals are stored over time in the organs, muscles, and brain, not the blood, so blood tests won't reveal them."

Hyman retested Dardia and found that he was overloaded with mercury as well as lead. Genetic tests also revealed a single nucleotide polymorphism that makes it harder for his body to clear toxins.

Hyman and his team created a rigorous detoxification program to help Dardia clear the heavy metals, after rebuilding his gut and his immune system so his body would be strong enough to tolerate it. "You can't just randomly detoxify or people get very sick," Hyman explains. "But you can remove mercury and lead safely in a controlled therapeutic environment."

At the Cleveland Clinic, Dardia started a supportive regimen of supplements and cleaned up his diet. His army physicians prescribed supplemental testosterone to help with his dysregulated hormones. And after four years of struggle, he started to feel better.

"It was like a fog was lifted off of me," he recalls. "My speech, mental clarity, finding words, task organization, all that stuff . . . all the people at work noticed: 'Hey, you're different. You're switched on.'"

RISK ASSESSMENT

One might assume that combat represents the greatest existential threat to military personnel, but most face a range of health hazards that are far less visible. These include hormone disruption from toxins emitted by munitions and burn pits, gut dysbiosis from prophylactic antibiotics used to protect against malaria, and tissue damage from parachute jumps and routine hikes with 70-plus-pound rucksacks.

Service members frequently suffer brain injuries from external assaults, such as traumatic knocks to the head and exposure to blast pressure waves, as well as internal forces, such as neurotoxins. Chronic pain can be a partner to all of these.

The basic conditions of military life will test the limits of any healthy person. "On average, we sleep around five, five and a half hours at a time," explains Captain Bryan Stepanenko, MD, MPH, IFMCP. "And, in a deployed setting, these soldiers may be up all night and trying to sleep all day, with mortars, rockets, or people working where they're trying to sleep."

Stepanenko is an active-duty family physician at Fort Bragg in North Carolina. Trained in both conventional and functional medicine, he believes that despite the many health challenges soldiers face, there's a lot they can do to prevent damage — and heal it when it occurs. This requires the right perspective.

GOING DEEP

In complex cases involving chronic pain, which are common in the military, a comprehensive case history is a vital tool. There's typically a threshold event, Stepanenko explains, after which someone will say he or she has "never felt well since."

"There are the emotional and the psychological stressors, but then there are the physical stressors," he notes. "You need to understand how much stress this body had handled already, because that tells you how resilient it may be, or how close that threshold might actually be."

A soldier he calls "Jones" (not his real name) is a case in point. Jones enjoyed a happy childhood and was active in various sports, though persistent tonsillitis meant he had to take more antibiotics than the average kid. He enlisted in the army in 2000, and seven years later was deployed to Afghanistan, where he was placed on prophylactic doxycycline, as are many deployed service members, to protect against malaria.

His job involved monitoring burn pits, which the military uses in the absence of civic sanitation services to dispose of batteries, Styrofoam cups, medical waste, plastics, computer parts, and other trash. Usually ignited with jet fuel — which contains benzene, a known carcinogen — these pits emit a stew of potent airborne toxins comparable to those encountered by 9/11 first responders.

Eight months into Jones's deployment, his health began to suffer. It started with gut problems and acid reflux. By 2008 he was suffering from chronic sinusitis and treating it with frequent courses of antibiotics. The following year, under intense stress while training for a Special Forces qualifying course, he required emergency gallbladder surgery after executing a parachute jump wearing nearly 200 pounds of equipment.

This led to still more rounds of antibiotics, all of which were depleting an already-stressed microbiome. Jones also had trouble sleeping and suffered constant musculoskeletal pain.

Then, after deploying with the Special Forces in 2012, he suffered a minor TBI that earned him a Purple Heart. It also broke him.

"He sustained four knockouts and 40 mild TBIs prior to the straw that broke the camel's back, which was driving a heavily armored vehicle over an IED," recalls Stepanenko. "It didn't flip the vehicle or anything crazy, but it was enough to where he bumped his head while wearing his helmet and he said he was 'never the same since.'

"He had sustained exposure to antibiotics for antimalarial prophylaxis. He had sustained exposure to burn pits multiple times. He had been exposed to multiple blast overpressure events in training and on deployment, and had sustained all those head injuries. But that IED explosion was the threshold."

In 2014 Jones was found unfit for duty after nearly 15 years of service.

A case like this could easily puzzle a conventional physician. That a minor head injury would be a breaking point doesn't make sense on its face, yet many healthcare providers don't have the time to learn what a body has already handled.

They do their best with what they have, and that often involves prescribing drugs for symptoms. (The Department of Defense spent an estimated $967 million on pharmaceuticals in 2017.)

By the time Jones found his way to the Cleveland Clinic in 2016, he had been placed on 44 different medications. His gut was swollen. He was in constant pain and routinely experiencing uncontrollable rage. He was anxious and depressed and contemplating suicide.

Learning what had preceded Jones's head injury, Stepanenko says, helped providers put his crisis in context. Not only was he devastated by his medical discharge from the army, which cost him his mission and his community, he was also suffering from runaway inflammation from brain injuries and gut dysbiosis. He had a "brain on fire."

Jones's treatment began with an elimination diet, followed by a ketogenic food plan. His gut health improved dramatically when he avoided wheat and sugar. He received testosterone-replacement therapy because his injured pituitary gland had diminished production of the hormone. He adopted relaxation techniques and began practicing archery. He lost weight, his bloating disappeared, his anxiety and depression eased, and his cognitive function improved.

Within three years, he was off most of his medications. Chronic pain and occasional bouts of rage remain ongoing challenges, but even these are gradually dissipating.

Without understanding the root causes for his

symptoms and receiving the tools he needed to heal himself, Jones would likely have continued to suffer from runaway inflammation and neuroendocrine dysfunction. The conditions would probably have worsened, possibly costing him his life. The drugs he'd been taking to control his symptoms were not enough. Yet recovery was possible for him; he just needed a different set of tools.

RUNAWAY INFLAMMATION

Brain injuries, toxic exposures, and gut dysbiosis produce a broad range of downstream effects that are typically intertwined. All can trigger runaway inflammation and systemic health problems.

Based on his own experience, Dardia worries that PTSD, while a genuine concern for many service members, is too often used as a blanket diagnosis when underlying conditions for mental-health issues might actually be physical.

"You can't fix a problem unless you frame and identify the problem," he says. "If you're a person who has all these things going on and you're just told that you have these four letters [PTSD], well, what the hell are these four letters?"

Chronic stress is itself inflammatory. When the

body's sympathetic nervous system is in fight-or-flight mode, the pituitary gland signals the adrenal glands to release cortisol. It's a healthy hormone in the right dose; the body needs it for energy, alertness, and inflammation control.

But when the nervous system gets stuck in the sympathetic mode, as it does for many service members, the rest-and-rebuild parasympathetic system never kicks back in. The adrenals eventually give up their high alert and stop producing cortisol. Energy flatlines and inflammation skyrockets.

Chronic inflammation is often a central feature of chronic pain. For Henri Roca, MD, who treats pain patients at the VA hospital in Little Rock, Ark., addressing inflammation is a key tenet of his protocol. He also strongly emphasizes the importance of self-care for patients and empowering them to heal themselves.

"Self-care skills give the greatest chance of pain resolution," Roca says. His patients learn to drink anti-inflammatory bone broth, which can help reduce the need for pain medication. They learn that brightly colored vegetables reduce inflammation, and that it's important to avoid sugar, fast food, and other inflammatory fare. They're taught gentle stretching techniques to address musculoskeletal issues.

And, crucially, they learn to give and receive support with other people in group medical appointments, a strategy that is central to Roca's approach. The strongest motivator for a disengaged patient, he says, is "the stories of other patients who have successfully reengaged with their lives and accomplished a degree of pain resolution and acceptance."

EACH ONE TEACH ONE

Marine Corps veteran Elijah Sacra is one such pain patient, and he has dedicated his postmilitary life to helping other injured service members recover their health.

He and his fiancée, Clarissa Kussin, run Warrior Wellness Solutions (WWS) in Durham, N.C., where they offer functional-medicine health coaching to active-duty service members and veterans. This includes dietary strategies to improve gut health and reduce inflammation, rehabilitative exercise, and restorative yoga and mindfulness practices.

Sacra learned the value of a lifestyle approach to managing chronic pain firsthand in 1993, when he fractured three vertebrae in his neck. "The culture of the Marine Corps at the time was 'take some Motrin and let's go.' I continued to do exercises with my arms being numb," he recalls.

Like many service members, he powered through it. But when he was honorably discharged and took a desk job in 1996, his spinal pain grew more severe. He soon changed course, pursuing a new career as a rehabilitative exercise physiologist.

As luck would have it, his first client came with a list of complex health issues that compelled Sacra to explore all the factors that contribute to a healthy recovery. That path eventually led him to study at the Institute for Integrative Nutrition (IIN) in New York City. The first military veteran to enroll there, he found himself in a strange new world.

"I'd never heard of smoothies; I'd never heard of wheatgrass," Sacra recalls. He was still eating fast food at the time. But that began to change when he met Kussin, an IIN health coach, holistic personal chef, and meditation teacher.

In 2009 Sacra launched WWS with fellow Marine Corps veteran Alvaro Matta, and Kussin soon joined their team. "We were teaching juicing, smoothies, and some rehabilitative exercise and yoga," he says. Sacra and Kussin attended the Functional Medicine Coaching Academy on scholarship.

The nonprofit has since provided health coaching to hundreds of service members, as well as their families and caregivers. Clients have routinely weaned themselves from their meds, lost weight, and even returned to active duty, all with the help of the dietary and lifestyle interventions they learned from WWS's health coaches.

The team remains available to coach its clients for the rest of their lives, should they find themselves struggling with weight gain or medication. Healing complex illnesses is an ongoing process.

THE RIGHT TOOLS

The Pentagon already recognizes that whole-person care is a good fit for service members. The army's 2016 Move to Health and the VA's Whole Health for Life initiatives place the patient at the center of the treatment model and emphasize the importance of nutrition, sleep, exercise, mindfulness, and social support. Sacra serves on a VA research advisory panel and a chronic-pain and opiate-addiction study committee.

More than 50 Department of Defense clinicians are currently certified in functional medicine. A range of integrative treatments — including acupuncture, chiropractic, biofeedback, yoga, and mindfulness — are now available to service members and veterans within the military healthcare system. Battlefield acupuncture has become a standard form of treatment for acute and chronic pain.

Still, functional and integrative services aren't widely used at this point, and many service members aren't aware of the available resources. Dardia, Stepanenko, and others are working to change that.

Dardia volunteers with TFD as a VA-certified recovery care coordinator to help connect people with unfamiliar integrative services. With Hyman, he's created a pipeline for SOF to get treated at the Center for Functional Medicine. He and Stepanenko have presented on root-cause medicine to clinicians and military leaders.

Stepanenko continues to blend functional medicine into the care he provides for patients on post, and he counsels soldiers on how to protect their health during service.

"I give probiotics to guys when they go on deployment. I tell them, 'Take your doxycycline and this. When you go over there and start breathing the air, drinking the water, and eating the local meat, take detoxifying chlorella, vitamin C, and modified citrus pectin. Drink plenty of water and make sure you're having bowel movements daily.'"

Dardia now deploys with what he calls his "force

field" supplements: glutathione to support detoxification, fish oil for inflammation, n-acetyl cysteine to support lung health, and vitamin D to boost the immune system. He also packs his own high-quality paleo protein bars as one alternative to the Meals, Ready-to-Eat (MRE) rations served in the field. "I haven't eaten an MRE since 2006," he says.

That doesn't mean Dardia's immune to new health challenges. He returned from a recent deployment with severely inflamed lungs and strange skin growths. But because he understands how his body interacts with his environment, he had the team and the tools he needed to recover. (This time they included a course of antibiotics and intermittent fasting.) Nothing surprises him anymore. He's ready for what comes.

"Everyone I know who is resilient has always had a contingency plan," Dardia explains.

If the military's present interest in whole-person health continues to grow, such contingencies— with nutrition, lifestyle, and social components— may eventually become one of its best defense strategies.

Dardia looks forward to seeing it. He knows that studying the "operational environment" is vital to solving any complex problem, including complex illness. In survival situations, knowledge is not just power.

NATIONAL SUICIDE PREVENTION HOTLINE

1-800-273-8255

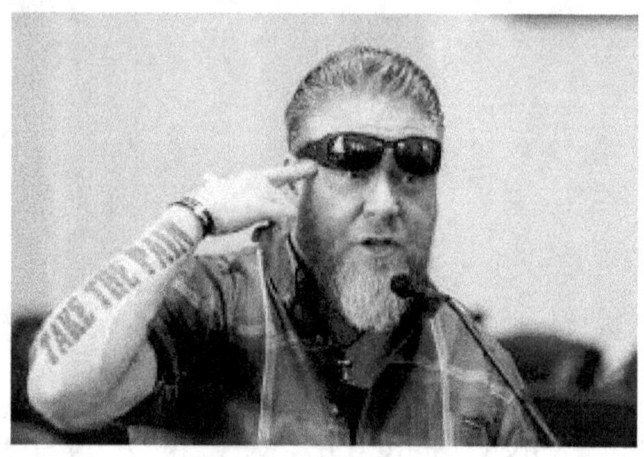

About Boone Cutler

Boone Cutler is an author, speaker, multi-media director, War- fighter Rights leader & Warfighter advocate with the distinct honor of being the first combat veteran from the current war to be a nationally-recognized, radio talk show personality.

Boone wrote his Iraq War-inspired autobiography, *Voodoo in Sadr City* (2010), during his two-year convalescence from wartime inju- ries at Walter Reed Army Medical Center during the Neglect Scandal of 2007. Those two years proved to be foundational to Boone's activism on behalf of Warfighters. Boone began writing his Iraq War-inspired journal during his combat tour in Iraq where he was deployed as a psychological operations specialist (PsyOp'er) to Sadr City, a sector of 2.5 million Shia Muslims, where he and his team were assigned to turn the psychological tide of the residents against Muqtada al-Sadr and his Mahdi Militia.

As team leader for the four-man psychological operations squad, Boone designed and implemented PSYOP campaigns that involved the following routine behavior: 1) influencing

Iraqis to sabotage the planting of IEDs, 2) influencing Iraqis to identify the murderers and rapists among themselves, 3) advocating for maligned Iraqis falsely imprisoned, 4) illustrating stories that best exemplify democracy to select groups of Iraqis and monitoring when and where those stories were repeated throughout the population, 5) reinforcing the positive behavior of Iraqis who helped their fellow men at great personal risk, 6) minimizing the fallout of Shia-Sunni racial tension by the strategic planting of messaging that routinely confused such concerted efforts, and 7) offering strategic advantages to tribal leaders for encouraging local cooperation with American forces.

Boone also has been active in messaging and advocacy work stateside both locally and nationally, his most public advocacy work being for Warfighters. Boone's most outspoken message is that the alternative to polarizing political climates in America is Warfighter leadership which is based upon volitional and self-sacrificial service towards a unified end across the entire cultural spectrum. He converges all of his efforts on law- makers who advocate on behalf of the Warfighter community 1) by bringing justice to civil rights violations and 2) by unifying a diversity of industry influencers within the civilian community towards this end.

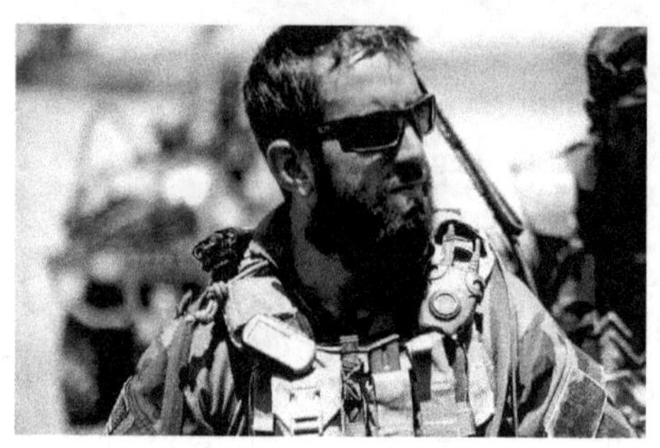

About Geoff Dardia

The Task Force Dagger Foundation Health Initiative Program started with Geoff Dardia, a SOF community member, in 2013. His story started like many others: he was "banged up" physically, mentally, and emotionally. Facing divorce, medical retirement, deep depression, and suicidal ideation, he refused to accept the standard of care and refused to believe a large portion of his symptoms were "all in [his] head."

Geoff sought care outside the conventional medical system. He started a transformational health experience that he later continued with the Cleveland Clinic Center for Functional Medicine, the flagship clinical care and research facility for the Institute of Functional Medicine.

This experience not only showed Geoff what was driving his conditions and causing his symptoms, but it also empowered him to address these root causes and protect himself from exposures inherent to the Military Operational Environment.

Ever since his healing experience in 2013 — in true force multiplier fashion — Geoff has been recruiting diverse professionals and advocates who share his Mission, Purpose & Focus. Their work through the Health Initiatives Program continues to empower others in the community and build the case for taking a Person-Oriented Medical Approach to caring for our soldiers and special operators.

The Brotherhood doesn't end after injury
illness, ETS or retirement.

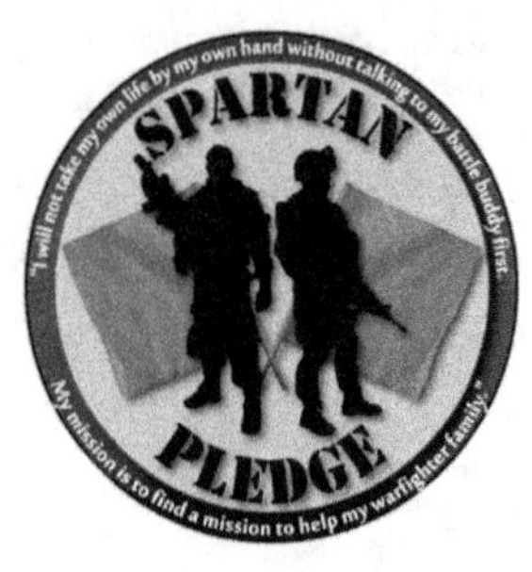

The Spartan Pledge

"I will not take my own life by my own hand without talking to my battle buddy first.
My mission is to find a mission to help my warfighter family."

TAKE THE PLEDGE TODAY!

facebook.com/The SpartanPledge/

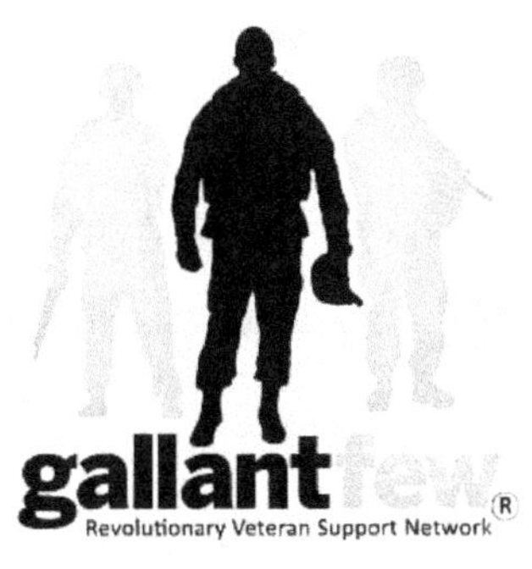

GallantFew

The core focus of GallantFew is one-on-one mentoring by a veteran with a veteran. We share lessons learned on active duty, but traditional transition doesn't share transition lessons learned. We want to change that, and we want to prevent veterans from becoming isolated and frustrated. You may feel that your thoughts, feelings and emotions are unique to you, but they aren't. We exist to facilitate a peaceful, successful transition from military service to a civilian life filled with hope and purpose.

READY TO GET STARTED?

GallantFew.org

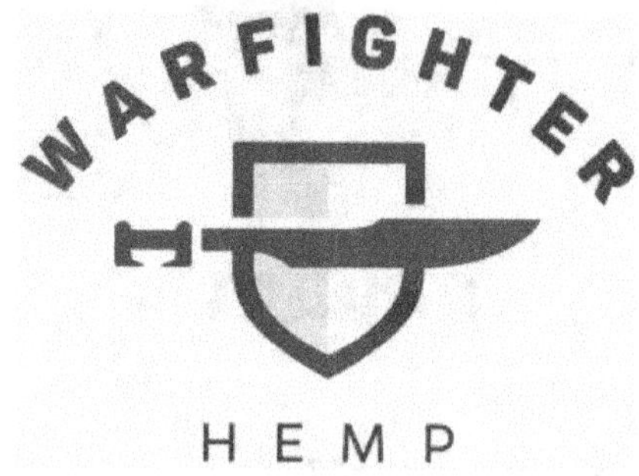

Warfighter Hemp

Warfighter Hemp provides our nation's veterans with an organic, non-addictive, non intoxicating means to improve the overall quality of their lives.

MADE FOR VETERANS BY VETERANS

warfighterhemp.com

American Addiction Centers

American Addiction Centers is the leading provider for addiction treatment nationwide, specializing in evidence based treatment and mental health care.

CALL US AT 888.342.0219

americanaddictioncenters.org

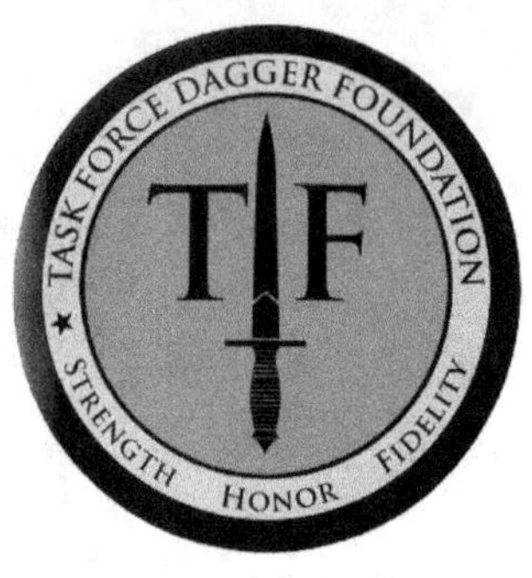

Task Force Dagger

Task Force Dagger Foundation provides assistance to wounded, ill, or injured US Special Operations Command (USSOCOM) members and their families. We respond to urgent needs, conduct Rehabilitative Therapy Events, and provide next-generation health solutions for issues facing our service members. We are a rally point to combat Traumatic Brain Injury (TBI), Post-Traumatic Stress (PTS), and environmental exposures.

SEIZE THE MOMENT AND LIVE LIFE!

taskforcedagger.org